How to Go On a Paleo Diet:

The Nutrient-Rich Eating Solution for Energy, Clarity, Clear Skin, Improved Sleep, Higher Immune Function and More

Summary

The purpose of this guide is to help you understand everything you need to know about how the Paleo diet works. This includes taking a look at how it can be run, what you should be eating and what you should not be eating. You can also learn from this report about how to stay active while on the diet and what you can do to keep yourself on the diet. You will also learn about what your body might feel like while on the diet. This book will help you to understand everything you want to know about this popular diet and how it can be as beneficial for you as it can be.

Table of Contents

Disclaimer and Terms of Use: Effort has been made to ensure that the information in this book is accurate and complete, however, the author and the publisher do not warrant the accuracy of the information, text and graphics contained within the book due to the rapidly changing nature of science, research, known and unknown facts and internet. The Author and the publisher do not hold any responsibility for errors, omissions or contrary interpretation of the subject matter herein. This book is presented solely for motivational and informational purposes only.

Diets and Their Importance

A healthy diet is critical for your life. You need to make sure that you focus on only the right foods when it comes to staying healthy. The problem though is that it's a challenge to do this when you take a look at the foods that are out there today. It might be easier for you to lose weight if you go back to basics just like what the cavemen did.

It sounds like an unusual idea but it's true – the Paleo diet is a truly unique diet that can help you to lose weight. It will not only make you capable of living a healthier lifestyle but it will also help you to avoid the harmful things that you might get out of foods these days.

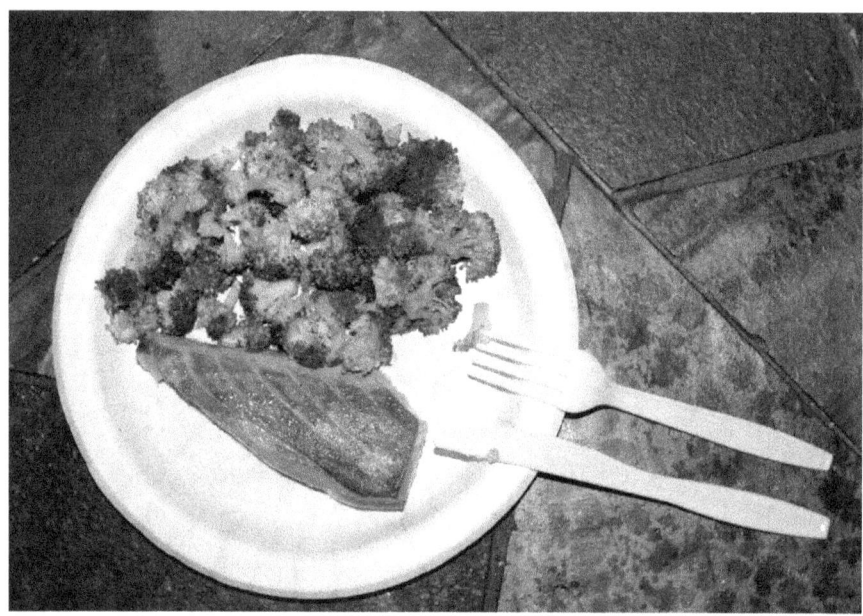

From Gluten Free Tube

What is the Paleo Diet?

The Paleo diet is one of the most interesting weight loss solutions for you to use. It is a kind of diet that focuses on foods that might have been eaten by hunter-gatherers in the past.

Hunter-gatherers in the Paleolithic Era, which is believed to have occurred about 10,000 or more years ago and as many as two million years ago, were forced to survive during that time with a number of foods that were found in nature. This often involved not only harvesting foods from the ground but also foods from animals that had existed alongside these humans at the time.

It is a very unique diet not only because it involves focusing on foods that would have been eaten by our ancestors but also because it may end up improving your life. Scientists have found over the years that many hunter-gatherers in this time had never suffered from chronic diseases or illnesses like the ones that people today often suffer from. It is a unique point about the diet that adds to just how valuable it could be.

In fact, it even puts an emphasis on how certain foods were not commonplace while on the Paleo diet. This includes many processed or refined foods that were clearly not around tens of thousands of years ago.

Let's be honest for a moment – when you think about cavemen you obviously think about things like hairy men, long hair, hunting dinosaurs, rudimentary wheels and the like. However, one thing you might be forgetting about is the way how cavemen had to work with a natural diet back then in order to actually survive for as long as they could have. The results of the diet may have proven to be useful to help them last much longer than expected. The big difference between them and you is that you don't have to be at risk of being hunted down by a creature that is at least ten times as large as you are.

The concept of the Paleo diet is easy to understand – **if the food you are looking at is something that someone from that far back in time could not have eaten then you should avoid eating it altogether.** It's as simple as that and should make it easier for your body to feel its best.

The biggest part of this diet is the key concept that many believers in the diet have followed. **Humans back in the Paleo era were known to have muscles, were agile and had an easier time with being more athletic.** The same obviously cannot be said about the average human in today's society.

Naturally, there are people out there who would say that the Paleo diet is a silly idea because the average person these days is living longer than ever before. That is true but the big question is whether or not the body is really taking advantage of a healthy lifestyle.

People are only living longer because they have access to more health care services and medicine. The odds are very good that someone in the Paleolithic Era that used the Paleo diet everyday probably would have lived longer than the average person would today if that person had access to the many health treatments that people have today.

Now is the time to see just how this diet can work for you. This is made with an interesting process that is made to keep anyone from gaining weight and to even give your body a stronger build after a while.

How It Works

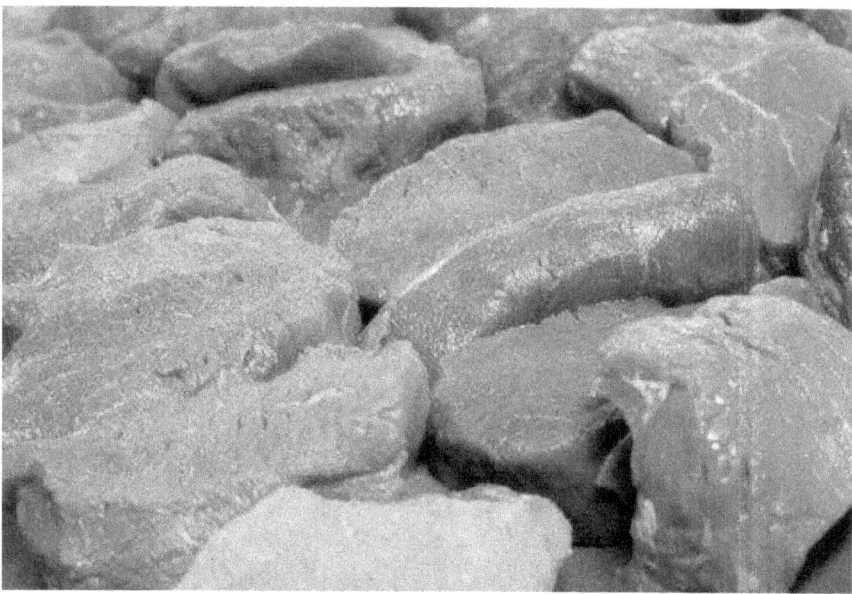

It's as easy as watching for healthy meat. (source)

The process of using the Paleo diet is very easy for you to understand. This involves a number of critical points to help you out with sticking to the diet:

1. First, you have to prepare your foods with the right items in mind. This includes scheduling meal plans ahead of time. The key is to determine what foods are sensible to eat based on what would have been available during this older time in history.

2. There is also the need to avoid consuming foods that were not around back then. You can learn more about what foods you should and should not be using in the next section of this guide as well as the kinds of foods that might sound healthy but are actually going to do more harm than good while you are on the diet.

3. The key is to eat when you are hungry. You should not be eating anything if you don't feel hungry. In fact, the diet rewards those who engage in intermittent fasting, a procedure that involves skipping a meal on occasion while making sure that you do not eat more than needed after you get back to a regular eating habit.

4. You then need to focus on a healthy exercise routine. This might be used to keep your body active and to make it more likely to burn off any excess calories or fats that you have added over time. It also works best if you keep your body under control without too much excess energy.

5. You should make sure that you keep your body hydrated as well. This includes making sure that you consume pure water to make your body a little more active and less likely to suffer from fatigue.

As you can see, the steps that have to be used when getting this diet used are not all that difficult for you to work with. It makes the diet more sensible.

Is It For Everyone?

This can be useful for anyone who wants to lose weight and stay healthy. In fact, people who want to lose at least twenty pounds could take advantage of the Paleo diet. It should make the weight loss process a little easier to manage.

Also, it works well for those who want to eat a good diet that features a variety of foods. It can be easier for you to lose weight with a healthy arrangement of natural food than it would be for you to just eat an extremely limited palate of foods or to just eat a bunch of expensive meals that have been prepared for you by some weight loss company.

Of course, this diet is not necessarily for everyone. There are a few people who should avoid using this diet:

1. People who are adverse to consuming meat for moral or ethical purposes might want to avoid this diet. The diet will involve plenty of meat because it is made with protein and less carbohydrates so you can build more muscle mass over time. (Interestingly enough, many stories you might read online about people who have used the Paleo diet are from former vegans who found that this worked better than their old vegan lifestyles. This doesn't mean that every single one will be comfortable with even thinking about this idea.)

2. Anyone who is concerned about dairy deficits might also want to avoid the diet. While it is true that many of the leafy greens involved in the diet do contain calcium and other dairy-related nutrients, the risk to some people suffering from extreme bone loss issues could be dangerous.

3. People who require grains to help with staying regular might want to avoid this diet too. The diet does restrict the use of grains. The effects of fiber and meat might support the body just as well as grains could but it's still a risk to think about for some cases.

4. Anyone who isn't willing to go along with the restrictions on the diet should avoid the diet. This diet is much easier to use than others but at the same time it might be tough for some to live with due to the rules that come with it.

5. Some people might not be able to afford the diet due to the cost involved with getting meats and other special foods prepared while on the diet. It will more than likely be more affordable than one of those special twelve-step programs with massive food packages that have to be bought but it's still more expensive to follow this than to just stick with the foods one is already familiar with.

A Special Note About the Kidneys

One critical part of getting into the diet involves seeing how your kidneys are functioning. This is because many of the foods that are used in the Paleo diet include purine. This is a compound that cam be broken down to form uric acid.

The excess amounts of purine in the body can be removed from the body through the kidneys as uric acid. This should help you out with keeping healthy.

However, a person with unhealthy kidneys may not be able to process the purine over time. This can cause gout or even kidney disease to develop at times. Therefore, you might need to get your kidneys examined and tested to see if they are healthy enough to actually process all the purine that you will be using while on the diet.

Talk With Your Doctor

This diet should work well but just make sure that you talk with an appropriate nutritionist before getting into the diet. Only a nutritionist can definitely tell if you need to go with this diet and if you are safe for it. It's all to make sure that you are fully aware of what is going on with the diet and that your body will have a positive response to it.

As you will see in the next part of this guide, there are many foods that can work well for your dietary needs. These foods can help you out with keeping yourself healthy and controlled.

Basic Pointers to Focus On

Foods for the Paleo Diet

The problem with so many diets is that they involve several restrictions relating to what you can and cannot eat. These restrictions are very annoying and tough to live with but at the same time they must work in order to get a diet to run right. It's especially problematic when you consider how some diets have extreme caloric restrictions or focus on only one food above all else that you could be using.

Fortunately, the Paleo diet involves a large variety of foods for you to choose from. You can take advantage of many foods in a large variety of categories. Here's a look at some of the foods that you can use while you are on the Paleo diet. **The choices you have proven that there's something for just about everyone on this diet.** You don't be easily bored when you are on it.

Meat

You can use a variety of meats in your diet. Beef, lamb, pork, sheep, rabbit and many others can be used here. These are all naturally occurring meats that should help you out with keeping your body healthy and under control.

You could even go along with organ meat if you want to. This can include such meat options as the kidney, heart or liver. You should probably avoid the brain due to its high cholesterol content but other than that the options you have for consuming animal organs are impressive to see.

These meats can also include proteins to keep your body healthy. Proteins are needed to make it easier for your body to build a healthy tone without adding more fat than needed.

You can also use poultry in your diet. This has less fat in it and might work well for you if you aren't comfortable with some of the other meat-based options on the diet. You can go along with chicken, turkey or duck among many other poultry meats.

These meats can all work provided that they are not impacted by anything that might add to caloric contents. These include things like salts, peppers, frying procedures and many others. The meat must be pure and unadulterated because that is practically what our ancestors would have eaten. Remember, you should avoid trying to eat anything that was prepared in a way that didn't exist back then.

It's especially important to use **grass-fed** meat. Grain-fed meat can be harmful to your body. Grass-fed meat will be leaner and healthier for you to use. In fact, most types of organic meat products come from grass-fed sources.

There are times where you might not be able to get this kind of meat though. Fortunately, you can always go with **lean meat cuts** while adding coconut oil or clarified butter to the mix.

Remember, the key is to think about handling your meats with all sources in mind. These include meats from the **air** (chicken, duck, etc.), the **land** (lamb, pork, beef) and, as you will see in the next section, the **sea**.

Fish

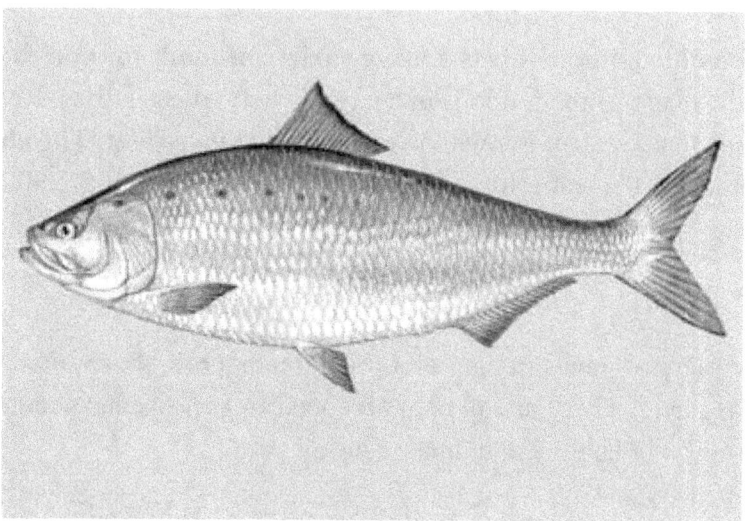

Enjoy an American shad on your diet.

Fish can be used in your diet. It's true that fish has some fats but these are healthier fats that have been found to help you out with weight loss needs. These include omega-3 and omega-6 oils. They are fats that are known to improve your body by keeping old toxins out and by removing old saturated fats that might have gotten into your body over the years. In fact, it can be easier to get these oils through fish than it might be to just use a simple supplement capsule.

You can go with all sorts of fish in your diet. These include fish like tuna, trout, salmon, cod, haddock, anchovies, herring and grouper.

You can also go along with shellfish. This is a kind of fish that is protected by a shell or other coating. You obviously have to remove the coating or shell in order to take advantage of it but the choices you have are amazingly varied. You can take in crab, lobster, shrimp and oyster options.

This can work well but **you should only go along with fish if you are not allergic to any fish-related products**. You can stick with meats instead but the key is to think about your general health and how you will respond to fish if you want to go on this diet.

Eggs

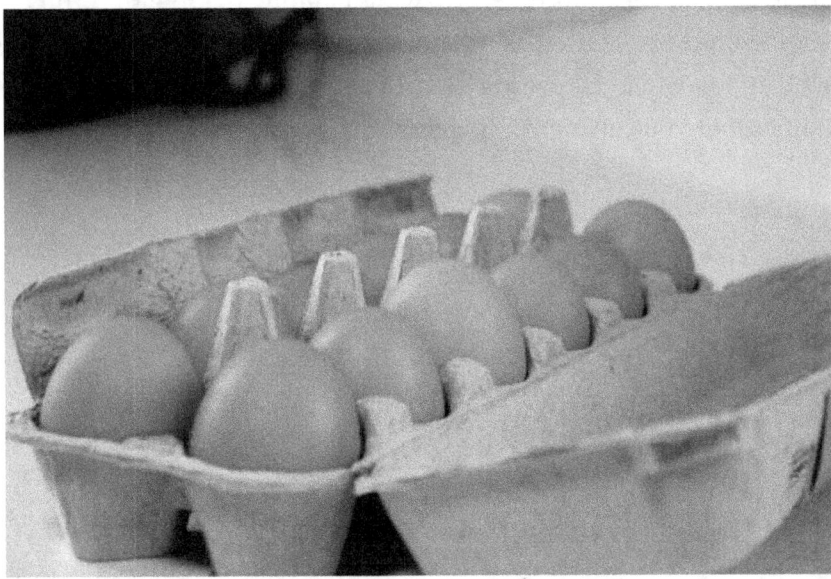

Use eggs in your diet. (source)

Eggs can work in your diet. These include eggs that come from different poultry-based animals. Eggs are capable of providing your body with choline, a substance that is used to help you get your heart controlled to keep the molecules that harm blood vessels down.

It is true that there are some egg allergies. However, **most people outgrow their egg allergies as they become adults**. Therefore, you might have an easier time with handling eggs if you are older in age.

Of course, you can always go along with a plan that only involves egg whites or egg yolks depending on what you want to get out of it. Just make sure that you only work with actual eggs and not egg substitutes. Trimming off the white or yolk parts of eggs should not be all that hard for you to do.

Fruits

Fruits are not only capable of improving you immune system but are also naturally sweet without any artificial sugars being added. The fruits that you can use include apples, oranges, bananas, pears, grapes, pineapple, coconuts, figs and many others.

There are no restrictions on the fruits that you can use either. Now it is true that some of these fruits might have fats in them like bananas. However, they should be easy for the body to use because the fats are organic in nature and should not be as likely to stick within your body as other processed fats that you might have been using before getting into this diet.

The best thing to do is to eat fruits carefully without going overboard. Fruits work well as a snack but they should not be used as often as vegetables. This may come from the natural sugars that you would be getting out of these fruits. This is in spite of the strong nutrient quantities that you can expect to get out of fruits.

Vegetables

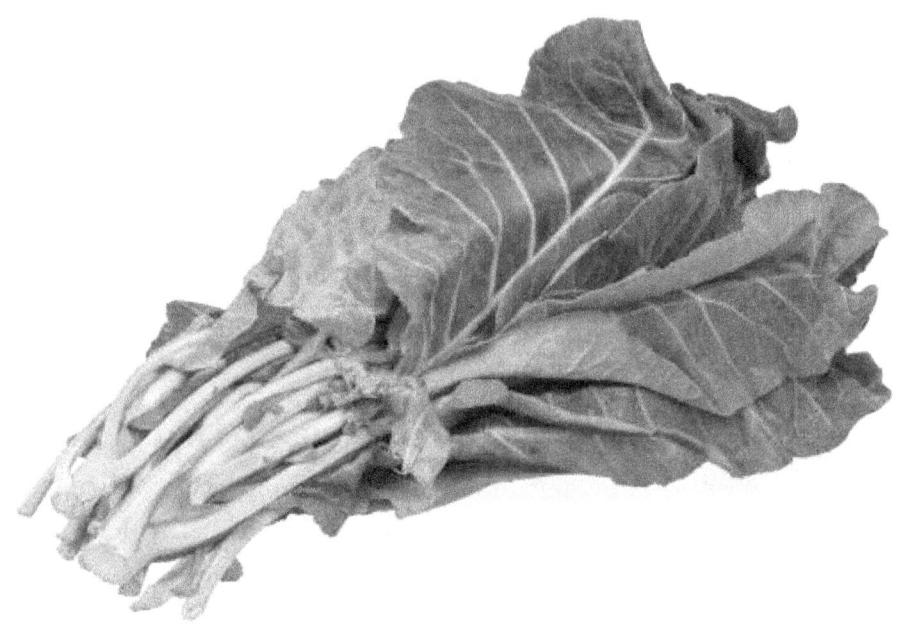

Collard greens can be used as vegetables in your diet. (source)

The vegetables that you can use in this diet are able to help you out with improving your body's ability to use fiber, calcium and other critical nutrients that you need in your diet.

Leafy vegetables are the most popular options to find. These include cabbage, lettuce, spinach, turnip greens and even mustard greens.

Root vegetables are also popular choices. These are vegetables that grow underground. They have been harvested by people for millions of years. Some of the vegetables that you can use here include carrots, radishes, turnips, beets and artichokes among many others.

Even squash can be used among vegetables. This includes winter squash options like butternut and acorn squash but also summer options like zucchini and yellow squash.

You can use these vegetables in either a **cooked or raw** form. This can be according to what you might personally prefer.

What About Herbs?

Herbs may also be used in your diet. These include choices like thyme, parsley, basil, rosemary, sage and dill. They can be used in small amounts to make something a little more enjoyable for your diet. They can naturally add to the flavor of your diet.

Don't Forget Spices

Some of the herbs that can work in the diet can be used as natural spices. In fact, you can use many of these spices to liven up your foods if you feel that they are not enjoyable enough for you. This is important because many of these spices include ones that have been used for generations in many diets.

The spices that you can use include ginger, garlic, fennel, black pepper, vanilla and nutmeg. The key about these spices is that they have to be naturally occurring and have been prepared in a safe and natural fashion without any additional materials.

Just be sure that the ones that you do use are controlled carefully. You should not be using spices with excess amounts of sodium in them. Salt and other items that contain sodium will only end up delaying your progress.

What About Water?

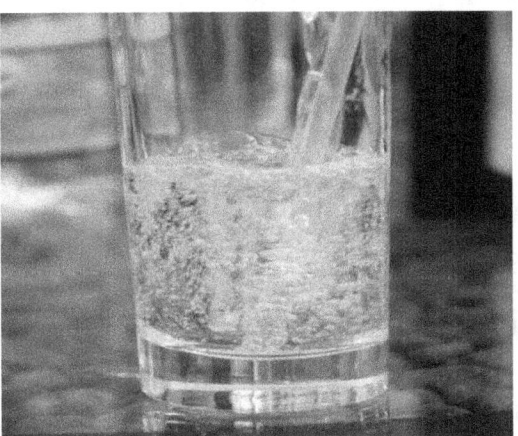

Water can truly work wonders on the body. (source)

You definitely have to use water if you want to go places on this diet. This is needed not only because it is naturally occurring but also because it can remove the old wastes that you have put in your body over the years.

You clearly have to find water that has been fully treated and cleaned without any salt or sugar ingredients. Pure water is the best way to go.

It's particularly helpful to go with a standard plan for handling water. This standard plan should involve working with about six to eight regular glasses of water each day.

You could also use coconut water or even organic green tea. They are options that have come from nature and could help you out just as well while on your diet. These are completely optional choices to go with but they may still be beneficial to your body.

Can Oils Work?

Oils can be used while you are on the diet as well. You have to clearly focus on oils that are naturally occurring if you want your diet to be successful. Olive, avocado and coconut oils are useful options to work with, for instance.

You should still be very careful when using your oils. You can use them for things like flavorings that can go over cooked meats or even a salad. This should make it easier for the oil to be noticeable without going overboard while using it.

Using Fats Right

You also need to see what fats you are getting out of these foods. You can work with one of three different types of fats from the right resources:

- Saturated fats should be controlled carefully. You can use them with coconut oil but they should be kept at a minimum for your safety.

- Some types of animal-based fats can work well only if they are from healthy animals. These include fats like lard and duck fat.

- Fats from oils can also work well if they are kept at a minimum too. These include olive and avocado oils.

You have to make sure that these fats are used carefully if you want your diet to work out right. This is all to keep things working without adding harmful fats that could potentially keep your diet from being run as well as it should be.

Stick with Clarified Butter

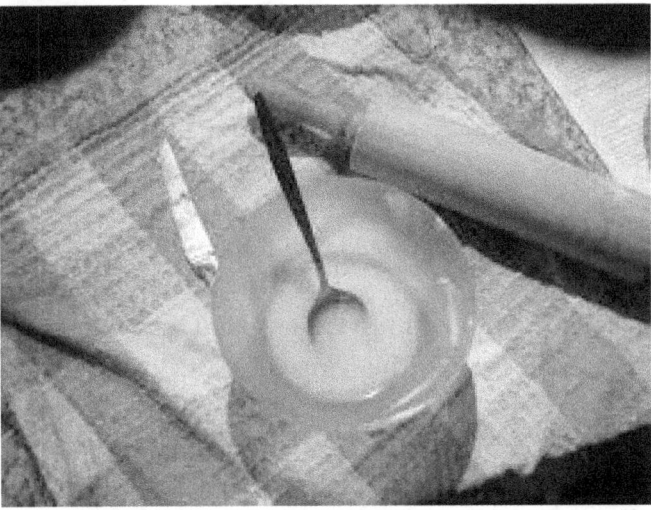

Clarified butter is a unique option. (source)

Butter may work on the Paleo diet if you are careful with it. It has to be prepared with natural procedures instead of with loads of salt like what some companies have been using in recent years. An idea to choose here would be to work with clarified butter. This is known as ghee in some cultures.

Clarified butter is milk fat that has been taken from butter and separated to where the water and milk solids are taken out from the butterfat. It can work with a more controlled approach to your diet.

You can easily find clarified butter in containers. However, it can also be made by melting butter and letting its contents separate from each other. This will allow the water in the butter to evaporate while solids on the surface are cleared off as needed. The milk solids will be stuck at the bottom while the butterfat is poured out.

Foods to Keep Away From

There are some foods that must be avoided when taking advantage of this diet. These foods include ones that clearly were not around back in the days of the caveman. There are also some foods that might have existed at the time but should still be avoided because they are not ones that might have been prepared for use in a natural manner.

You should particularly watch what you are doing with these foods because they are made with all sorts of harmful ingredients. These include several things that clearly were not around in the caveman days. You must make sure that you keep yourself under control and stay away from these harmful items in the diet.

Dairy Items

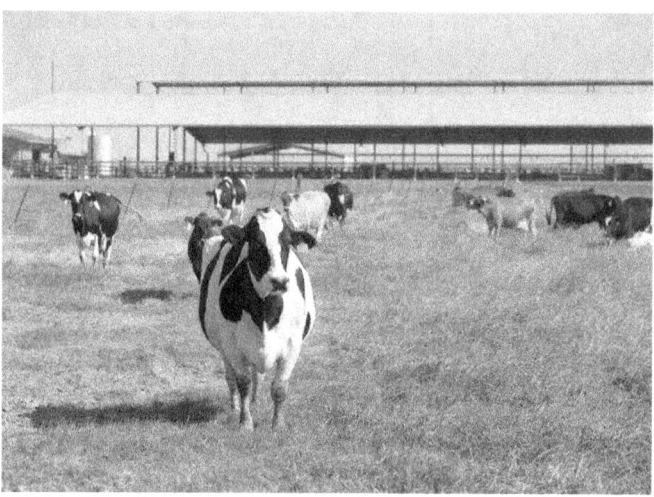

Cows weren't domesticated back in the day. Why use their items in your diet? (source)

There were no procedures involving cultivating dairy products from animals in the Paleo era. This is because they weren't being domesticated at this point in time.

There's also the problem with dairy items on today's market being subjected to all sorts of abuses. Many items are heavily processed as they are prepared for consumption. There are also many items from animals that can be subjected to all sorts of hormones and artificial treatments just to try and get them to taste better.

Grains

The concern about grains is that they can contain gluten, a substance that is known to keep the body's digestive system from working properly. There is also the concern about how a majority of grains in today's society have been heavily altered with additives to get them all growing right.

You particularly have to avoid rye, barley and oats if you want to keep your diet going well. It's also best to avoid corn.

It's especially important to understand that many of these grains are made with high carbohydrate contents. This could be harmful to your diet due to how they will make it harder for your body's metabolic procedures to run well.

Sugars

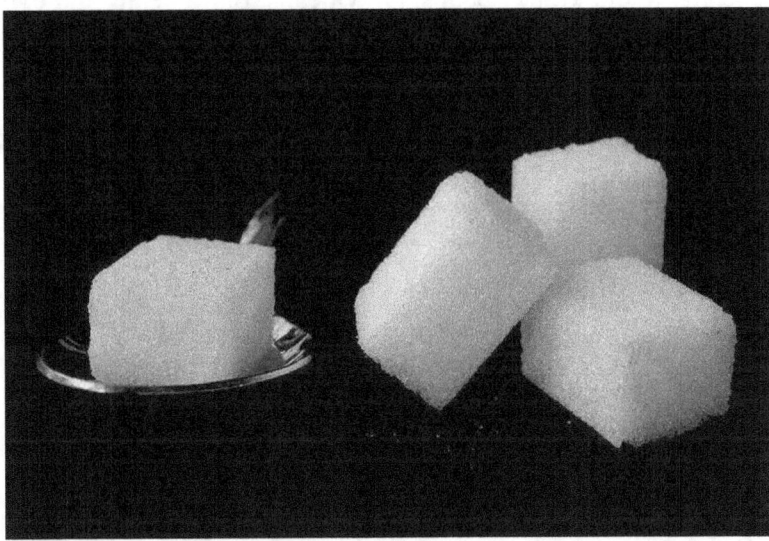

These small cubes are more harmful than you think. (source)

Sugars can be harmful because they will slow down the body's ability to take advantage of its weight loss functions. They may even contain artificial materials that can weaken cells around the body. It's especially the case for sugar substitutes that supposedly give you the taste of sugar without all of the health issues that come with actual sugar.

Trans Fats

Trans fats are dangerous because they can be found in many foods that have been heated up to the point where molecules around their bodies will be changed to where the fats are going to cause damages to cells around the body. They can even introduce new free radicals into the body.

In addition, trans fats can cause cell membranes to weaken. This can damage the body and make it feel worn out.

You need to make sure that the foods that you eat do not have trans fats and that you prepare them the right way without adding trans fats. This is to keep you from suffering from the risks that come with them.

Legumes

Legumes like peas, beans and peanuts can also be harmful. They can prevent the body from absorbing critical nutrients. They might also disrupt the body's digestive system just like grains can. You have to avoid these in this diet. This is even in the event that you see some options that are made with safe organic materials in mind. They are still going to be tough for you to digest over time.

You should especially avoid kidney beans, navy beans, pinto beans and even black beans while on the diet. These are some of the more harmful kinds of peas that you might run into while eating.

Farm Fish

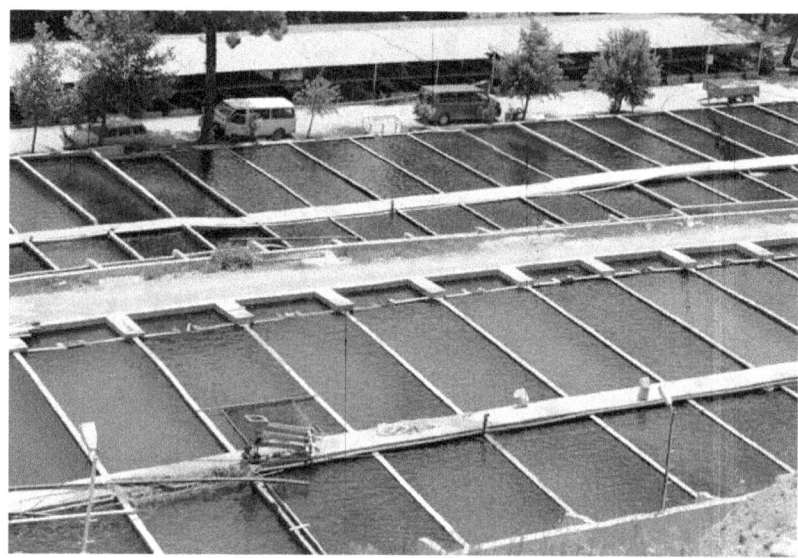

Do you really want to eat fish from a place like this? (source)

As mentioned earlier, fish are good for the Paleo diet. However, farmed fish are dangerous. Farmed fish are ones that were prepared in a farming environment where people commercially raise fish and treat them with different nutrients and substances in order to get them to spawn faster than what they might do while in the wild.

Products from fish farms can be dangerous because many of the products used in fish might contain traces of mercury. This could prove to be devastating to your diet. Therefore, you should **stick with fish that has come from nature and not from a farm.**

Certain Drinks

You have to be cautious when using different drinks on the diet. You have to avoid sugary drinks and drinks with sodium in them. These will end up causing bloating and fatigue.

It's especially important to avoid alcohol during the diet. This includes all beer and wine products. Even "alcohol-free" products have to be avoided. These technically contain trace amounts of alcohol with the average alcoholic content by volume being less than one percent. It's obviously safer than traditional alcoholic beverages but it still has alcohol nonetheless and therefore should be avoided.

Even "diet" drinks with zero calories or sugars should be avoided. The chemicals in the artificial sweeteners used in these drinks can be harmful to the body.

The Wrong Oils

While it is true that some oils can work while on the diet, there are also some oils that can prove to be dangerous on it. You need to avoid oils like sunflower oil, peanut oil, canola oil, soybean oil and even corn oil. Margarine and some shortening products like Crisco also have to be avoided while on the diet.

You have to be aware of these oils because they will come from some of the many foods that you clearly have to avoid. As mentioned earlier, you do have to avoid peanuts on the diet. Even the oils that come from peanuts can be just as harmful to your diet as the peanuts themselves. You have to be very cautious if you want to keep your body healthy and running well so you can stay healthy and focused.

Don't Drink Your Food

You particularly need to avoid any kind of "meal replacement" food when getting on the diet. This can include something like a nutritional shake.

It's true that these shakes and other replacement fluids can help you get nutrients. However, they also contain enzymes that might be hard for the body to use. They can also contain more sugars than what you can afford to use.

The most obvious thing about avoiding these is that they are drinks that were clearly not around in the caveman era. You have to focus on a more sensible approach to eating by working with actual food and not with something that claims to be a suitable replacement for whatever you are trying to eat.

Packaged Weight Loss Food

There's always going to be the temptation out there to try packaged foods that promote weight loss. These are often prepared in things like bars, frozen meals and drinks. These might sound great but they can actually be tough to work with.

In addition to these not being real foods that were around back in the early days of man, the problem is that these foods are prepared with assorted preservatives, salt and chemicals to make them taste better and to keep them safe as they are being transported from one place to the next.

There's also the issue of how the foods in question are boiled in order to keep them safe and sterile. This might make the foods easier to consume but it also makes it harder for the foods to have the right nutrients that you need for your weight loss goals. Therefore, you clearly have to avoid these foods if you want to actually get some kind of weight loss result out of your diet. This is in spite of the promises you'd hear when seeing what benefits you could be getting out of your meal.

Now that you know what you should and shouldn't be eating, you can get started on the next part of having success on the diet. This includes being as active as you can be.

Keeping Active

You have to keep a healthy and active lifestyle going while you are on the Paleo diet. The odds of you staying healthy while on the diet will be important to see because they relate heavily to keeping your body running well so you won't have to worry about any problems with your body not doing anything.

Part of this involves working with not only activities of a moderate level of intensity but also exercises that relate to what our ancestors might have done in the past. It's interesting to think about how people in the past worked out with rudimentary practices and were able to stay healthy. You can practically do the same today even if it involves working with more modern technology to make it a little easier for you to stay as active as possible.

Evolutionary Fitness

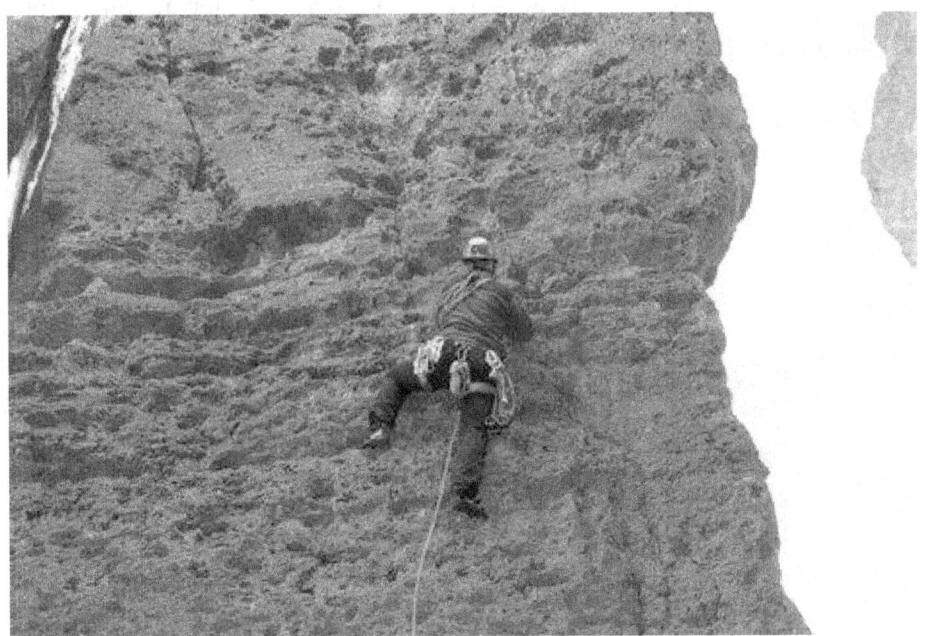

Rock climbing is a thrilling activity. (<u>source</u>)

An interesting part of using the Paleo diet involves evolutionary fitness. This is a part of fitness involving exercise actions that your ancestors might have done hundreds of thousands of years ago.

These exercises were essentially done with endurance in mind to make it easier for the body to be a little more active and likely to survive in more conditions. Today you can use them in safer environments but the key is still the same. You'll be able to work well with all of the muscles that you need to get taken care of in order to have the best possible body that you could be getting.

Many of these exercises involve the following to help you keep active and ready to do anything that you can. These involve completely natural forms of exercise but they can be performed with modern technology:

1. Running on tough surfaces; you could do this barefoot if you wanted to

2. Lifting heavy items

3. Rock climbing

4. Sprints and other running activities on an incline, preferably an uphill one

These are all activities that are believed to have been done by people back in those days with survival in mind. You can easily get on the road to a healthier life and a more active lifestyle if you go along with a diet plan that involves these activities.

Of course, you can always get into these exercises with things like a treadmill or a climbing wall. As you will see in the next part of this report, you can also do this with a strong series of weights. Either way, it should be easy for you to get better results out of a workout when finding a way to stay healthy and under control.

Strength Training

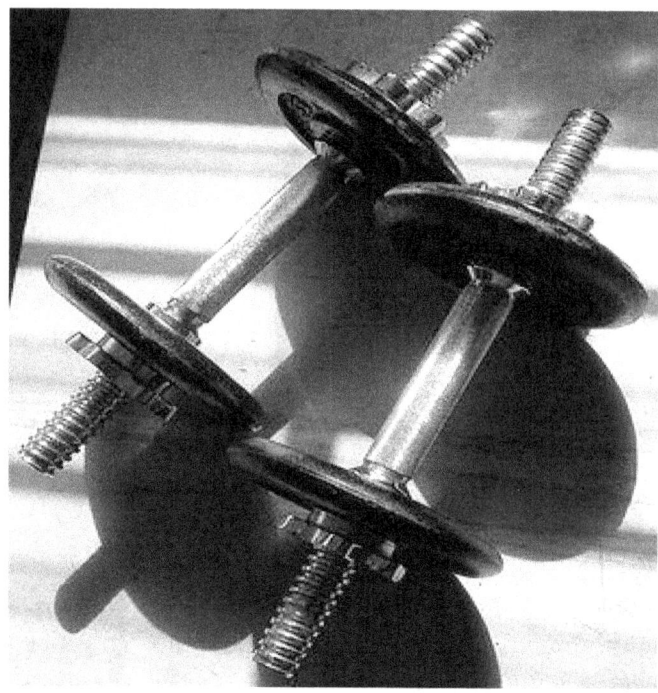

Lift your weight away (source)

Strength training may also be used in the process of keeping your body healthy. This can be done with the intention of building muscles. You can use lunges, push-ups and even squats with weights on your body to help you build muscles.

This concept has been a popular staple of the Paleo diet for years. It is believed that many cavemen had built strength by lifting heavy objects. I'm not saying that you should be grabbing a giant boulder and try to throw it someplace but you should at least work with some kind of strength training plan. This is assuming you go with something a little more realistic and sensible.

You can work on practically any muscle system in your body. The key is that you will be building lean muscle mass while keeping fats from being stuck in those areas. This should make you both healthier and stronger. It should give you the extra energy and muscle that you have always wanted to get out of your body.

In fact, this can be done with not only weights but also with pressure from your own body. Traditional calisthenics can be used over time to help you out with exercising your body and making it more likely to burn off calories and fats in the long run. It should help you to stay as healthy and under control as possible.

Just be sure that you watch for how much weight you are handling at a given time. You need to work with only the right amount of weight based on what you are comfortable with using. This is to make sure you don't end up straining yourself.

You can easily add to the weights that you use over time. The key is to just be comfortable and advance to more weight when you are actually capable of doing so. If you don't do this then you could be at risk of hurting yourself after you try to lift more than what you really can use at a given time.

What About Cardio?

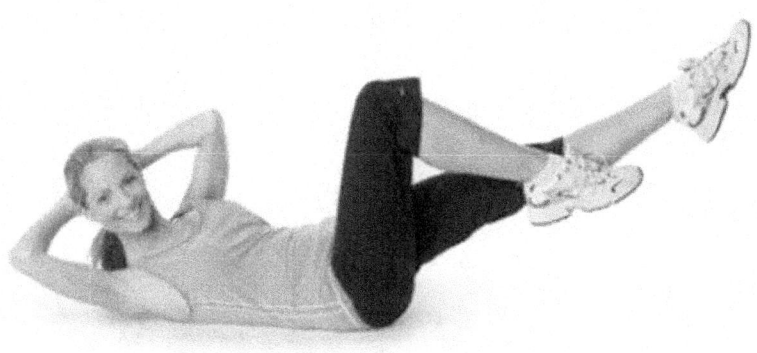

Cardio exercises work well if you use them carefully.

Cardiovascular exercises could work well but you have to watch what you are doing here. This includes making sure that you avoid working too hard when getting into these exercises. It's true that many people like to feel the burn that comes with these exercises but that doesn't mean you have to work with too much or too little effort just to get the workout used the right way.

It's a good idea to use a healthy and controlled pace when walking or when doing any movements that involve plenty of effort on your part. You do not want to do more than what your body can really enjoy because it might end up being a little too taxing on it. You have to make sure that you still have energy leftover for all of the other things that you want to do over the course of your day.

In fact, working out harder than needed can be dangerous because it might cause fatigue. Also, it might add to the pains that you could experience in your body. These pains can make it easier for you to try and possibly stray off of your diet. This is the last thing that you want to do when you are trying to lose weight.

Overall, you should strongly consider these moves if you want to keep your body as active as possible. These should be used well to help you out with keeping your body running well while on your diet.

Remember, you have to make sure that your diet is controlled well enough. You have to do this the right way if you want to keep from gaining weight during the diet. The foods that you have to choose from might be limited but they are at least varied in terms of what you could choose from.

What to Expect From the Paleo Diet

Note: The results that you will get out of the Paleo diet can vary according to who you are and how well you can use the diet. It's best to consider using this diet for about two weeks to see how well your body responds to it. You should be able to get a few benefits off of it but at the same time it might help you to see if you are likely to actually get even better results if you go along with the diet for a longer period of time.

Weight Loss

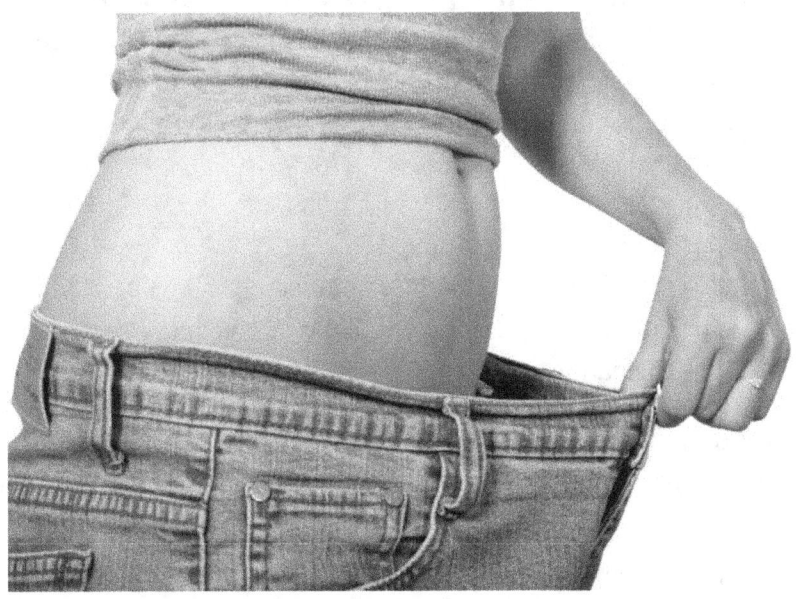

How much can you lose? (source)

There are many great things that the Paleo diet is capable of giving you. One of the best things involves the potential weight loss that you would be getting off of the diet.

You should be able to lose weight as long as you stick with the plan for the diet. This includes making sure that you stick with only the right foods and the right nutritional standards when handling the diet. Fortunately, the wide variety of foods that you can use on the diet should not make it too hard to work with.

You can lose **at least five to ten pounds within the first one or two months** after you get on the Paleo diet. This might not seem like too much but at the same time it will come from how you are eating healthier foods.

It's also safer for you to lose weight at this rate than it would be if you were to go along with a crash diet. The rapid nutrient loss and dramatic starvation that you'd experience during a diet like this could be harmful.

Of course, everyone is going to have different responses to the Paleo diet with regards to weight loss. These will relate heavily to four important things:

1. Your age; it might be easier for younger people to lose weight

2. Your personal genetics

3. Your metabolic rate

4. Your health as it already is

Of course, you could have **better results through a healthy exercise program and through portion control**. Keeping your dining portions from being as large as they could be and staying physically active should make it easier for you to lose closer to fifteen to twenty pounds in about two months after getting on the diet.

Energy Levels

The energy levels that you will experience while on the diet will be better for you to work with than what you had prior to the diet. You will have more energy because of the healthy proteins that you are eating.

In addition, the lack of artificial sugars in the diet and an extreme reduction in toxins from the diet should be used to keep your body functioning as well as it possibly can. You might have an easier time with keeping your body from being worn out easily. You won't be as likely to experience crashes either. This makes it all the more important for you to see how well the diet can be enjoyed.

Of course, much of this comes from the body controlling its eating habits to where you will not be likely to wear yourself out after eating. This could improve not only your ability to perform daily activities in life but also your ability to get a good night's sleep.

You need to use this diet to make yourself feel more active and under control. The diet is made to make you feel your best and to be more likely to stay up and at them with everyone else out there.

State of Mind

The mental benefits that come with going on the Paleo diet can be particularly interesting to see. You should be more likely to enjoy these points:

1. You won't be likely to suffer from serious issues relating to feeling tired. This could improve your attitude during the day.

2. You will also feel more productive with all that energy you will be getting. This should make you feel more positive about yourself.

3. The added focus that you get should improve the quality of whatever work it is you might do during the day.

4. It may even be easier for you to mentally focus on your diet at hand. Many diets fail because people forget to take a look at what they want to do with their eating habits. A better diet will help you to stay a little more active and under control so nothing wrong can happen.

Physical Improvements?

You might be amazed at the physical improvements that you will experience while on the Paleo diet. These relate mostly to how your body will respond to it over a period of time.

Improved Measurements

One of the best points about the diet is that you will have a better series of measurements around your body. These include measurements that have been toned down because you will have more lean muscle around your body and less fat tissue.

For example, you may be able to lose about one or two inches off of your chest in about one or two months on the diet. Also, you can lose two to four inches off of your hips. This is a part of the body that might be tough to do on your own but can be easily targeted while on the Paleo diet.

Less Bloating

Bloating occurs around the body when an unhealthy diet is consumed. This can especially be disruptive to your abs.

This is where the Paleo diet may come into play. The diet can help you to reduce bloating and get you to have flatter abs. This is thanks in part to the way how the diet is capable of providing you with natural sources of fiber that haven't been processed. It also helps you out with plenty of water and a dramatic reduction of salt in your diet.

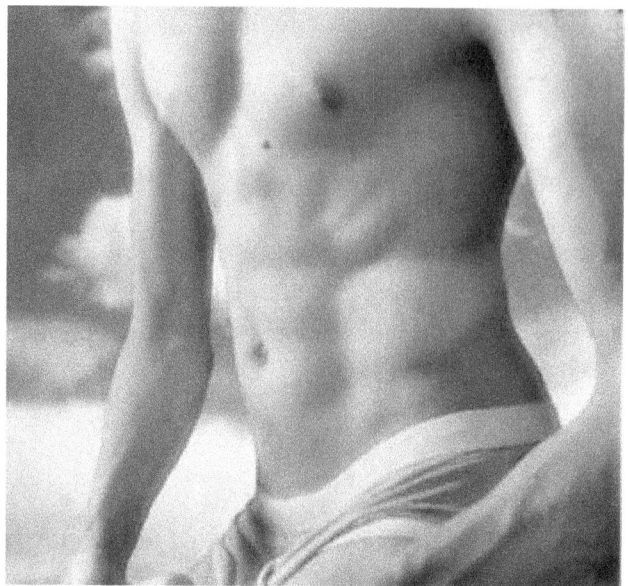

Your abs will look better without all that bloating. (source)

This should help you to keep the tissues in your abs from being worn out easily. It can also help you to get more defined muscles in the area.

Easy to Control Eating Habits

It will be easier for you to keep your eating habits under control while on the diet. Much of this involves how the diet will use foods that are filling and will keep you from wanting to eat more than you have to. This is especially the case when it comes to the water you consume and the natural fibers that you'd be getting out of your vegetables.

The filling nature of the diet should make it easier for you to keep you eating habits under control. This may make it easier for you to control your eating routine over time. It certainly gives your body something to look forward to in the long run.

Different Conditions That Can Be Improved

Many other positive things can occur when you go on the Paleo diet. Here are a few of these special positives:

Improved Breathing

The reduction in pressure on your body from unhealthy food might also be helpful for your diet. You should be able to correct many breathing issues including asthma and potentially sleep apnea.

Much of this involves how your body should be able to burn off enough fat over time to improve the ways how airways in your body are working. It keeps the body from suffering from obstructions that can cause snoring, sleep apnea and other occasion breathing difficulties to occur.

Issues with Allergies

Sometimes the regular diet that you are on might end up causing allergic reactions that can easily disrupt your life. This primarily comes from how so many foods that you would be consuming each day contain gluten and casein. These are two ingredients that trigger many food-related allergies.

The Paleo diet does not include many of the foods that might cause food allergies to flare up. You won't find nuts, wheat or milk on this diet.

Improved Digestion

Your digestive system will not suffer from damages from gluten when you go on the Paleo diet. This should keep your body active and more likely to burn off calories after a while.

In addition, the lack of lectin from grains in your diet will also be a big point of keeping your body healthy. Lectins have been known to get into the body's GI tract. This can keep the tract from being able to keep itself healthy and to repair itself as needed. The damages from lectins can be harmful but you can keep them from being prominent if you use a healthy routine with the Paleo diet.

Improved Hair and Skin Quality

The nutrients in your diet should make it easier for you to develop more hair. You hair will have a better shine to it and it will also be a little stronger. It might even be a little easier for you to grow hair in spots where it has been a challenge for you to actually get it going.

Also, the nutrients will be made to improve the quality of your skin. It will make your skin look alive and healthy after a while. This should keep you from suffering from too many issues involved with keeping yourself looking attractive.

A Better Immune System

The problem with so many foods these days is that they are laced with so many difficult artificial ingredients and flavors that they can make it harder for you to stay healthy. They can add to the toxins in your body, thus making it harder for your immune system to function properly. This could make you more susceptible to a number of illnesses.

The Paleo diet should make it easier for you to take care of your body and to keep these problems from being too dramatic. You can use this diet to help you out with losing weight from toxins being cleared out while also keeping the body's natural defenses a little more active over time. This is needed to help you with keeping yourself less likely to become ill after a while.

Reduced Pains

It's easier to suffer from pains around the joints if you are overweight. This is due to the added pressure that comes all that excess weight. Fortunately, the weight loss that you will experience while on the diet should make it easier for you to avoid the risks that might come with pressure.

Healthier Organs

You can also get your organs to feel better when you use this diet. This is thanks to the way how your organs will not feel too much pressure from fats in the body. There's even a benefit related to the way how the body can start burning off fats over carbohydrates for energy.

This benefit results from the way how your organs will begin to burn off fats that they have built up over time. These include ones that were not made for organ structures. It might even be easier for your liver and other critical organs for digestive purposes to be a little more open and capable of handling your body's activities.

As you can see, the effects of the Paleo diet can be very positive on your body. You should strongly consider this diet if you want to get the best weight loss results and feel better about your body all the way around.

Simple Life Changes to Ensure Success

Plan

You have to make sure that your Paleo diet plan is set up right if you want to lose weight with it and stay on the diet for a while. Many people who don't do well on the diet tend to be those who struggle with trying to get the diet up and running as well as possible.

There is a clear need to work with a few points to help you out with setting up a plan. A plan should involve working with a few simple steps.

What's in Your Cabinet?

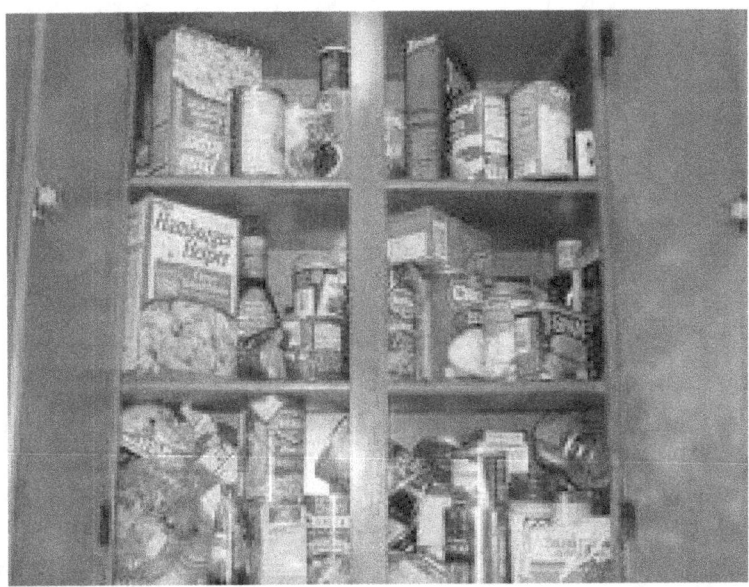

At least half of the things that are in this cabinet won't work in the diet. Clearing it out is the best thing to do. (source)

You need to make sure that you remove foods that are not in the Paleo diet from your home. This includes removing any products that appear to have been artificially processed. The key is to simply avoid all foods that have not appeared back in those times so you can make sure that you avoid the temptations that come with them.

What you do with the food that you clear out is up to you. For example, you can consider giving the food to other people in your neighborhood or even donating it to a local food bank that could really use it. Either way, the key is to make sure that you get everything that doesn't work on the Paleo diet cleaned out.

Besides, you'd be amazed at how much room you would create in your cabinets if you cleared out the stuff that you shouldn't be using while on the diet.

Consider Your Meal List

You then have to take a look at the meal list that you can use when getting into the diet. This may include details on the different kinds of foods that you can consume while on the diet. These foods will vary in terms of what you can and cannot go along with and should be considered carefully.

Keeping a Diary

You should make sure that you keep a diary running while on the diet. This should be used to list information on the following points:

1. When you were eating something

2. What you ate at the time

3. Any results in your weight loss plan

4. How you felt after eating; this includes whether or not you were actually hungry after you finished eating

The diary is used to help you out with not only recording what you have done but also to see how well you are going on the diet based on what you have been doing. The information you get out of your diary can prove to be effective and helpful for your weight loss needs thanks to how it will all be run with your general health in mind.

What Will Your Meals Be?

You then need to plan ahead of your diet by setting up an appropriate list of meals that you can use while on the diet. This list should include plenty of options to choose from while on the diet and can be arranged with individual times of the day in mind.

A good plan would be to set up a meal plan that can work over the course of a few weeks. This is used to help you out with figuring out what your meals are going to look like. These include different meals that feature different parts of the diet to keep you healthy.

Your meal plan should involve meals for breakfast, lunch and dinner. An appropriate snack may also be added in between lunch and dinner if needed. You should use this for a few weeks so you can prepare yourself as well as possible.

In fact, it might be easier for you to stick with the diet if you use a variety of meals on the diet. This should be prepared through a meal plan diagram to help you make sure that you are not going to become bored with eating the same things every single day while on the diet. You will not be likely to be bored by the diet if you focus on a plan with multiple kinds of foods in mind in order to keep your body healthy.

Remember, **this is all subject to whether or not you actually feel hungry.** You can always skip a meal or two during the course of a week if you do not feel hungry. Eating when you aren't hungry is just going to keep the diet from working out as well as it should be able to.

Set Time for Exercise

You have to prepare yourself after a while for exercise if you are to stay healthy. Your planning can involve setting up an exercise routine that involves a number of workouts each week.

You should schedule your workouts based on the times that you have available and what you want to do with them. This is so you can get your body prepared for all the exercises that you have to use while dieting.

Any Recipes You Can Use?

It's also helpful to see if you can find quality recipes relating to the diet. The odds are very good that you can find some recipes that include only the safest ingredients for eating while on the diet. This should improve your chances of losing weight and sticking to the diet.

These recipes may also be useful for helping you out with sticking to the diet by using only the right ingredients. It should make the shopping process for the diet a little easier to live with. Speaking of which, that is the next point that you should be taking a look at.

Shopping for the Paleo Diet

Shopping for the Paleo diet does not have to be a real challenge. In fact, you can easily get you shopping done once you have an appropriate meal plan set up. This should help you out with only the right ingredients and foods for what you plan on using while on this diet.

Of course, the foods that you will have to pick up should be very specific. This includes working only with foods like what you've already read about here. However, there are several other things that can be done in order to make it easier for you to shop for foods on the diet.

Organics are Useful

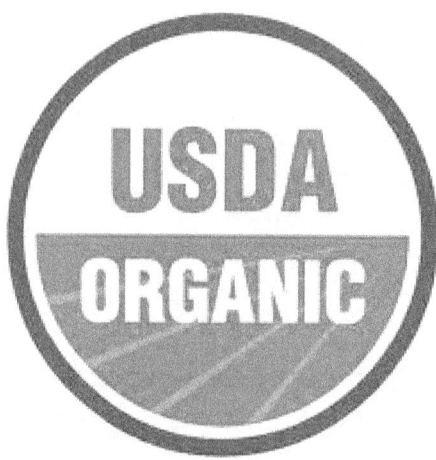

The USDA's official organic food certification label. (source)

First, you have to see that you are going along with organic products that have not been treated with artificial materials. One of the best options to find among organic products involves meat-based products that have come from grass-fed sources.

It particularly helps to see what labels are listed with regards to the certification that a certain product has gotten from an organization like the USDA. Groups like this can certify products as being organic based on how they are prepared and readied for people to use.

Always Check Labels

You should see what the ingredient labels are on different products that you buy. The odds are very good that something that has a bunch of artificial ingredients or some things that you have never even heard of will be off-limits during the Paleo diet. You always have to check and see what is included.

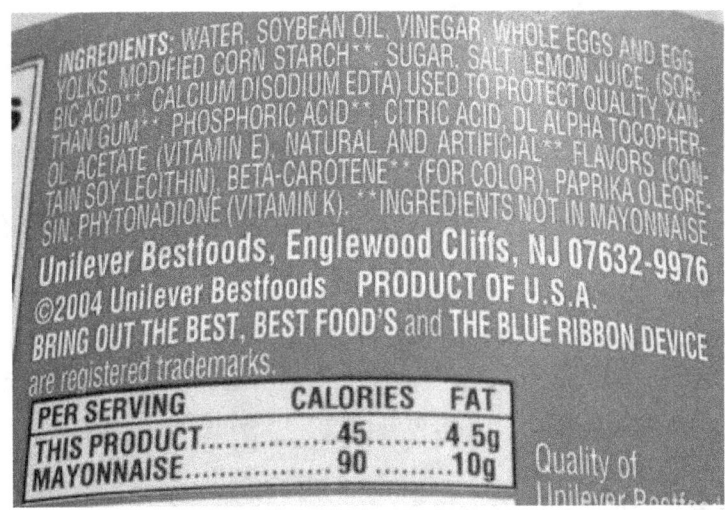

Always check on the label. (source)

The nutritional label can also help you to see how many calories come from something and any fats that are involved. This is to make sure that you get something with only the right fats and as little saturated or trans fats as possible. It's also good to see this in order to get an idea of how many sugars are naturally found in something that you are going to be using while on the diet.

Check Your Recipes

As mentioned just recently, you can have an easier time with planning for the diet when the best diet recipes are considered. You should keep your shopping list limited to whatever ingredients are listed on these recipes. This includes sticking specifically to different kinds of foods that were already listed on the recipes that you have found.

Always When Not Hungry

There is also the need to avoid shopping for the Paleo diet when you are hungry. It has been found from one study after another that shopping while you are hungry is a dangerous thing to do. It can make it easier for you to gain weight by buying more food than what you really need to get because so many foods will look more appealing when you are hungry.

This is especially problematic considering how so many markets and food companies get their foods displayed in a way to where it will actually make you want to eat something right now. You must control your diet by buying the foods you want when you are not hungry.

Ask Someone Else for Help

It might help you to stay on the safe side and ask someone else to shop for you if desired. This can be done by providing someone with an appropriate food list to use when shopping. It is a simple idea but it could be a real key to dieting success considering how it might be easier for a person who follows your instructions to get foods for you.

This could also help you to avoid the temptations that come with so many foods found in a market. Temptations can be very tough to control and can throw you off of a diet. Therefore, you have to protect yourself by avoiding them at all times even if it means having someone else go out to buy your food for you while on the diet.

Habits to Let Go Of

It's always tough to get accustomed to a new diet. This is especially if you have been so used to certain habits over a period of time. However, you will have to concentrate on a few things in order to make it easier for you to avoid losing time on the diet. Here are a few habits that you need to stop dealing with when trying to use the diet.

Controlling Breakfast

It can be a real challenge to enjoy your breakfast while on the Paleo diet. The truth is that you have to let go of habits relating to dairy products and cereal grains while on the Paleo diet. These are obviously not needed in the diet but it can also be tough for you to work with if you aren't careful enough.

You might have an easier time with getting through these pressures if you use a controlled breakfast that features appropriate meats that have been prepared carefully alongside a fruit or two.

Avoiding Sugar

You also have to let go of the habit of consuming sugar in your diet. Sugar is only going to hurt your chances on the Paleo diet due to the added pressure that is created on your body. You have to consider substituting sugary drinks with water if you want to keep your diet under control.

Remember, you might experience some withdrawal symptoms while avoiding sugar at the start. Keep reading this guide to learn how you can take care of these symptoms.

Excess Exercise

You need to work with exercise but you should avoid any exercise that might be strenuous or tough on your body. This includes avoiding excess cardiovascular workouts.

The key is to make sure your body is healthy and capable of handling the efforts that you are getting yourself into as you are trying to lose weight.

Sticking to Set Eating Times

While it might sound like a good idea in theory to stick with some very specific times for eating, you should make sure that you avoid the habit of eating at extremely specific times in the day. You should be eating when hungry and never when you don't have a real need for doing so. This is even if it requires you have to skip a lunch or dinner just to get in the diet. Remember, **your gut feeling for eating is the key to keeping on the diet.**

Temptations and Distractions to Avoid

Every diet has its own series of temptations and distractions and the Paleo diet is no exception. You could end up dealing with many pressures from outside sources to try and break off from you diet. However, it is not too hard to get away from these pressures if you know what you are doing when trying to keep yourself on the diet.

The Rewarding Process

You might think that you can reward yourself with a day off from the diet after a while. However, this is only going to make things harder for you to deal with because it will be easy for you to gain back weight that you have lost if you end up straying from the diet.

You clearly have to watch for what you are doing with yourself while on the diet. Be sure to avoid trying to reward yourself with any old food that you want to use. You really need to stick with the particular plan for handling food the right way.

Keep Your Mind Controlled

You simply need to politely decline anything that people try to give to you while on the diet. You have to easily control yourself and make it easier for you to avoid eating more than needed if you work hard enough with a healthy diet plan. Much of this involves working with your mind being controlled well enough to where you can avoid eating the wrong foods.

You should not feel guilty when declining temptations from others. Just remember that this is all for your own good in the long run.

Avoid Going Out While Hungry

You should make sure that you eat something in your diet before heading out anywhere. The key is to make sure that you are not hungry when heading somewhere. It will be easy to stick to your diet if you make sure that you don't go anywhere while you are hungry.

Being hungry while out of your home can be harmful because it will make you more likely to break off of your diet and eat something that you should not be having.

Don't Be Fooled By Advertisements

The final thing to do is to make sure that you watch for what advertisements for healthy foods might say. It's true that some healthy foods market themselves as being useful for Paleo diet users. However, this is not always going to be the case.

You have to check on not only the ingredients of something you are looking at but also whether or not there was any substantial processing involved with getting something created. This is important because sometimes something that might seem healthy might actually be harmful.

A good example of this came from the Wow Olestra chips that were released a while back. These sounded great in that they have fewer calories and fats but the problem was that they contained ingredients that were able to not only prevent the absorption of nutrients within the body but also ingredients that might disrupt one's bowels.

As you can see, something that claims to be a healthy option is not always going to be as cracked up as you might think it is. Therefore, you have to be extremely cautious when trying to get any kind of food like this to work in your diet. This is to prevent you from struggling with foods that might not be great for you.

Some Bumps to Expect with the Paleo Diet

The Paleo diet, like any other diet, is not something that is easy to get into right away. You can't just choose to go on the diet and expect your body to feel comfortable in just a snap. You have to focus on a few things with the Paleo diet in order to keep it running well.

Withdrawal Symptoms

Although the Paleo diet does include a much larger variety of foods for you to eat than some other diets, it is also one that forces you to stop consuming some foods that you have gotten used to. The process of getting away from these foods can be a challenge for some to work with though.

That's why it is so important for you to take a look at what you want to do with the diet. This includes watching for the cravings that you might have for foods that you are missing. It is a completely natural thing that might be problematic because you are so used to some of these foods.

What makes this harder is the way how you might be stuck with fatigue and anxiety from the diet. This is because your body will start to do things that you aren't used to feeling. It will start to burn off fat for energy purposes after a while due to the lack of carbohydrates that you'd be using.

Here's a short list of some of the withdrawal symptoms that you might experience when you start following the diet:

1. Fatigue

2. Headaches

3. An increased sense of irritability; this might be due to the lack of sugar that you would be consuming while on the diet

4. Aches and pains; they should not be too extreme to the point where where your body will not be able to move properly

5. Light-headed feelings and dizziness

6. Some dehydration; this might come from the body having an easier time with removing water after a while

You will probably end up experiencing these effects about one or two days after you start using the Paleo diet. In fact, they could occur midway through the first day in most cases.

Fortunately, it should not take too long for these effects to go away. You might expect the effects of these withdrawal symptoms to wear out in about three to five days after you start the diet. Everyone's responses will vary though; some people take longer to recover.

These symptoms might be tough to deal with but they can be controlled if you know what you can do. There are many ways how you can cope with these symptoms and even make it easier for you to stop feeling them after a period of time.

How to Cope with Symptoms

You should not have to be held back by these symptoms while you are on the diet. You can take control of these symptoms if you do a few helpful things while on this diet.

Eat Fat

You have to make sure that you eat enough fat while on the diet. This is to make sure that your body has more energy.

Of course, this fat should come from healthy sources like with organic meats. However, you can always add a tablespoon of coconut oil or avocado oil to help you out with keeping your fat intake up at the start of your diet.

The key is that fat will help you with getting energy so you will have an easier time with burning off sugar. This should help ease your body into this new stage.

Keep Water In Hand

The second thing to do is to make sure that you consume enough water while on the diet. The reason why this is needed is because a reduction in carbs in your diet can result in your body becoming dehydrated. Your body will be more likely to excrete fluids in your bowels when you lose carbs. Therefore, you have to get a healthy amount of water in your diet each day.

In addition, water can be used to fill your body up. This should keep you from feeling hungry after a while.

Don't Be Too Active at the Start

As mentioned earlier, you need to have a healthy workout lifestyle if you want to lose weight on the Paleo diet. However, you need to make sure that this new lifestyle is not used immediately. You have to get used to the diet before you can actually exercise to your heart's content.

The key is to keep from getting into any high-intensity workouts during the first few weeks of your diet. This is to make sure that your body can get used to what you are doing with the diet.

Consistent Eating Habits

You have to use consistent eating habits as well. These habits should involve working with regular meals without skipping anything.

The key of this is to make sure that your blood sugar levels are kept in check. Your blood sugar levels can be very shaky at the start of the diet. A regular eating regimen should make it easier for you to keep your body from feeling ill.

As you can see, the Paleo diet can be easy to take part in if you use the right strategies to keep the negative effects down. However, there are some times where the diet has to stop as you will see in this next part.

Signs You Should Stop

While the Paleo diet can be useful, the amount of weight loss that you can get off of it might be limited. You can experience results but after a while it will get to the point where your body has nothing else to lose off of the diet. This is where the risks that might come with the diet can really get in the way of keeping your body as healthy as you want it to be.

There are also some times where you might have to stop using the diet if only to keep your body from being at risk of serious damages as a result of it. Here are a few signs for when you should be stopping the diet.

Your Weight Loss Tapers Off

There will come a time in your diet when you stop losing weight on a regular basis. This might be easier for you to notice if you have been keeping an appropriate journal that keeps tabs on how well you are losing weight.

Your Desires for Food Change

There are times when you might start thinking about food too much. This could include having a sudden desire to look for sugary or fattening foods that contain fats that might be too harmful.

The reason why it might be best to stop at this time is because you could be more likely to overeat after a while. This could prove to be even more harmful than what you might have been experiencing already when trying to lose weight.

Your Sleep Habits Change

Sometimes you could suffer from poor sleeping habits if you suffer from a poor diet. The reason for this comes from how your dietary habits might involve different nutrients that might change dramatically depending on what you are doing during your diet.

The problem here is that your body will be more likely to suffer from a lack of sleep. This might add to your hunger over time and might even cause you to eat at times in the day where you really do not have a need to eat.

Following a plan to eat at the right times of the day based on when you are hungry is clearly the way to go when it comes to keeping this diet under control. However, you have to make sure you keep a healthy sleep habit going. If you are doing everything you can to keep your sleep habits working well but you still are hungry then that might be a sign that you are not doing well with regards to staying along with your diet.

You Have Concentration Changes

There are times where you might develop changes to the ways how you can concentrate on things. This might involve times where you are unable to focus because you are not getting enough nutrients in your diet. You need to control your Paleo diet experience carefully so you can avoid problems relating to your diet. However, you will also have to stop with the diet in the event that what you are going through is proving to be harder for you to enjoy than what you might have expected.

You Start to Feel Pain

Finally, you will have to stop with the diet if you have started to feel pains around your body while dieting. The pains that you might experience as a result of a diet should go away not long after you start.

However, there are times when your body will not respond to the Paleo diet or it will have done as much as it could for your body. This can result in your muscles wasting and wearing out after a while. You have to stay if you are dealing with problems relating to how well your muscles are responding.

You need to use these points when figuring out a way to keep yourself healthy while on the Paleo diet. Failing to control your body well could end up causing more harm. Going longer than needed while you are on your diet could also be problematic and risky for your long term health needs.

Habits to Adopt

It will be easier to go along with the Paleo diet if you use only the right habits for your diet and lifestyle. Here are a few of the things that you should be doing in order to keep yourself on the diet for as long as possible.

Make the Food Interesting

Sometimes people get tired of the same old foods while on the Paleo diet. They often want to go along with foods that are a little more exciting and easier to enjoy. Here are a few things you can do to make your foods a little more interesting and enjoyable.

Keep a Good Variety

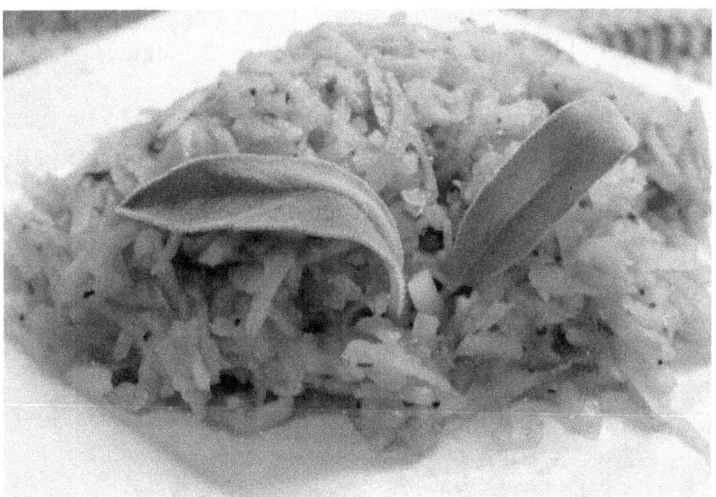

Sides like sweet potatoes can be useful for variety.

You have to start by making it a little easier for you to keep your foods under control. Part of this involves having some variety in your foods. You can do this by using a variety of options when getting your foods controlled:

1. Take a look at different side dishes that you can use alongside your meals. These side dishes are made to add to the overall experience of dining and can work well with practically anything that you have in mind. For example, you can use roasted vegetables, apple coleslaw, coconut bread or even an orange and cashew salad as a side dish.

2. Make sure your foods are as varied as possible based on your meal plan. This includes looking to see how foods on the diet are spread out based on when you will be eating them and that you are not going to repeat meals after a while.

3. It always helps to find desserts to keep you happy and comfortable when on the diet. Desserts like berries with almonds, bake bananas and even apple chips can be good to enjoy on the diet.

4. You can even make some Paleo diet editions of some long time staples to any diet. For example, you could go with a burger that does not have a bun on it. Of course, you have to make sure that the burger is made with grass-fed beef if you actually want it to meet the Paleo standards you have.

Make Sure Dressings and Toppings Work

You can use many toppings and dressings on foods. You can use healthy herbs and oils like what was mentioned earlier in this guide. These should add some flavor to whatever you are eating, thus giving you a little more experience with your food while keeping it from being bland. It might even work well if you think you are naturally adverse to some of the foods that you should be eating when you are on the diet.

You can use these well but you have to watch for how they are to be used. The goal is to avoid using them with too many things at the same time. You have to cover everything properly with only the right amount of toppings to keep it all healthy and under control.

Fun Ways of Keeping Active

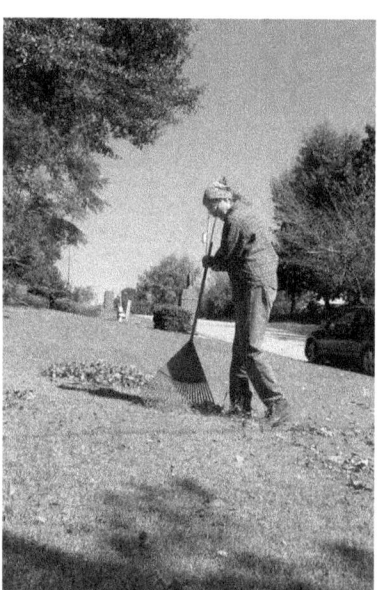

What seems like a chore actually does more. It keeps your body active.

You don't have to worry about the pressures that come with having to exercise all the time just to keep on the diet. You can easily have a better time with sticking to the Paleo diet if you think about some ways how you can keep your body active and under control.

Here are a few of the things that you should be doing in order to give yourself an easier time with keeping your body running well.

1. Exercise with a friend or even a family pet. It always helps to have someone alongside you while you are working out.

2. Make sure you use that extra effort when getting from one place to another. For example, using the stairs instead of an elevator while at work or at some other place is always a good idea. You can even choose to park a little further away from your office than what you usually do.

3. Play along with your family members if you have any. It's always good to throw the Frisbee around, for instance. It makes it so you can have quality time with your family members.

4. Water activities can always be enjoyable. These include not only swimming activities but also things like rowing or paddling.

5. Raking leaves or doing other kinds of yard work outside is also great to do. This is fun because it allows you to be closer to nature.

6. Feel free to find competitive leagues in your area that allow you to participate in sports of all sorts. These can include bowling leagues or even tennis leagues.

7. Find a local bike or walking path in your area. You could even consider going on one that you have never been on before.

The choices that you have to choose from are great to find when thinking about getting active. You can easily use these while on the Paleo diet to keep your body active while keeping yourself from being bored.

Involve Friends and Family

You need to get other people that you know to work with you while you are on the Paleo diet. It should make it easier for you to succeed because you can get others to support you as you go along the Paleo diet. You can go along with one of these strategies to make it easier for you to get others to go along with the diet:

1. Take a look at getting other people involved in the process of cooking meals for the diet. This might be enjoyable to some because the reward of eating what someone makes is always a great thing to find.

2. Talk to friends and family members about what makes this diet so unique. They might be more interested in helping you out if they are fully aware of what's going on with it and how beneficial it can be.

3. Try talking about the unique foods that can work on the diet. Sometimes it's easier to get people into the diet when they are aware of the unique options that work while on the diet.

4. Invite them along with you on different exercise activities. It's easy to get them into the diet if you work with enough encouragement through an active lifestyle.

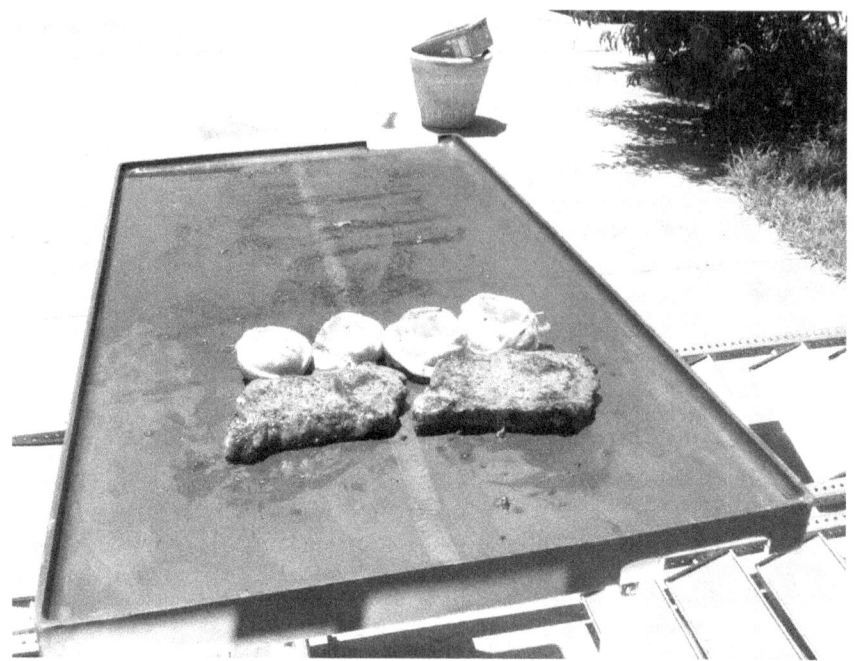

Cooking can be enjoyable for anyone.

5. One idea that might even be better would be to invite people over to see how you can cook things on the diet. This could be done to show people just how easy the diet truly is and how you can get it to run well no matter what type of food you are looking to get out of it all.

Reach Out to Paleo Enthusiasts

You would be amazed at the variety of places where you can find people who are easily interested in the Paleo diet. In fact, you'd come across so many people on a search engine that you'd have to tough time with keeping track of everyone one of them.

You should keep in touch with a good Paleo diet community. You can have an easier time with sticking to the diet when you are with a community that has the same goal as you. In fact, you might even learn more about the diet in the process if you learn from these people about what you could be getting out of the diet.

You can get in touch with a number of Paleo enthusiasts if you do a few things to make it easier for you to find them. Some of the ideas to use include the following:

1. Look for local meet-ups with people who are interested in the Paleo diet. You can learn more about the diet and find out more about what you can be doing when on the diet when you work alongside a group of people who are looking to become healthy like you are trying to do.

2. Contact different websites that might be dedicated to listing information on the Paleo diet. You can reach out through chats with other Paleo dieters and even exchange tips with them. The online Paleo diet community is much larger than what you might think it is like.

3. Check on recipe databases online to see what's around. You could share information with other enthusiasts about what foods you are using and how you can incorporate them into healthy recipes that work well on the diet.

4. Head out on exercise walks with others on the diet. You might get a good friendship or partnership going based on the diet you are on and the interests that you and your exercise partners are into.

These ideas can help you out because they may make it easier for you to enjoy the diet and to get the best results out of it in the long run.

One Step at a Time

Pacing yourself is important for any kind of diet. The Paleo diet is no exception to the rule. You have to do a number of things while on the Paleo diet to keep yourself under control and many of them involve making sure that you work with the right pace to stay healthy and under control when trying to lose weight.

You simply need to concentrate on keeping a steady pace by working one step at a time. You have to do this if you want to keep yourself from suffering from more pressure than what you can afford to use while on the diet.

The things that you can do while keeping the diet in check for you are important to see. You need to do the following in order to get the best results out of the diet:

Control Your Meals

You have to see that you control your meals while on the diet. This includes making sure that you focus on eating healthy foods that are natural and aren't processed in any way.

Much of this clearly involves sticking with a plan for handling meat and fish to make sure that you keep your body running right.

Progressively Remove Negative Things

The process of getting into a healthy diet can be tough for anyone to do. That's why you should think about removing the negative foods from your diet progressively to help you out with keeping your body safe.

Part of this involves removing legumes and grains over time and replacing them with meats. This should help you to get more protein among other nutrients.

Pay Attention to Your Body

Your body is the most important messenger in the diet process. You have to watch out with regards to what your body is trying to tell you when you are looking to lose weight. Much of this involves concentrating on a plan to consume only the right meals at the right times. Keeping a close look out on how your body is working is a key to making it easier for you to actually lose weight after a while.

You've got to observe all the changes to your body as you are on the diet too. These changes might involve your body experiencing sudden pains or even irritability. These are problems that can keep you from feeling active and need to be corrected if you want to keep your body under control on the diet.

Staying on Course

Staying on course during the Paleo diet can be a real challenge. Then again, you could say that for practically any kind of diet that you want to go on. However, many of the most successful people who have used the Paleo diet have done so for one to three years at a time.

You should take a look at what you are doing with your diet if you want to stick with it. Here are some handy ideas that you can easily use to stick with the diet.

Focus on Individual Meals

Don't feel the pressure of having to run with the diet for a while. You should simply stick with a plan that involves consuming food on a plate by plate basis. In other words, you have to pay attention to each meal you get as you get it instead of trying to stick with a plan that involves what you will have a month from now.

A good meal plan should help you to get an idea of what you will eat each day for a few weeks. That should be as far out as you can go when planning your diet. You should always treat the next meal you will have as if it were the most important meal that you'll have ever had while on the diet. It's all to keep things running carefully.

Always Use a Rotation

It's good to have variety in your diet. However, it also helps to have a few dishes in your regular rotation so you can go back to them as you see fit. These can include dishes that you have had in the past while on the diet and want to enjoy again because you thought they were delicious.

This can help you out by keeping a sense of familiarity with your meals. Familiarity is needed to help you out with keeping the diet running without any surprises that you might not feel all that comfortable about.

Prepare When Going Out

You have to be prepared for what you will be going to do when heading outside your home. It's especially important if you are going to be on a vacation for a certain periodof time. Here are some things to do with this in mind:

1. Try and prepare some meals a few days beforehand so you know you have stuff to eat while out of your home.

2. See if you can get foods that don't have to be cooked. Sometimes foods like fruits and vegetables for the Paleo diet can be used without having to cook them in any way. You can simply wash them to make them safe.

3. There are times where you might be encouraged to head to some place to eat out at. You must make sure that you research any spot that is going to be in the area you'll be at before seeing if you should go there. Try and check on the menus of these places if they have websites that you can look up. Check and see if they can adjust the foods that they prepare in accordance to your dietary needs as well; most places should do this for you if you just ask politely.

These are good things to do but the real key is that you have to make sure you are not going to make it so people who travel with you are going to get upset with what you are up to. The people you travel with should feel comfortable with what you are doing when heading places. It's easier for non-Paleo people to be frustrated when you have to make loads of changes. Therefore, planning ahead of time when you are going out is by far the best thing that you can do in order to keep your diet running as smoothly as possible.

Celebrate Milestones

You should reward yourself when you get to certain milestones while on the diet. These milestones can be great to achieve because they will show that you have been able to work hard on the diet and have avoided problems relating to how it is run.

Celebrating milestones is always a good idea because it encourages you to work as hard as possible to stick to your diet. It's also to make it so you will want to feel more positive about how your diet is going after a while. You can get milestones set up with a variety of different points relating to the following:

1. Completing an entire cycle on your meal planner without slipping off of it

2. Lasting for a certain amount of time while on the diet

3. Losing a certain amount of weight

4. Getting a better physical measurement around your chest, hips or other problem area you want corrected

The things you can do to celebrate one of these special milestones can vary but they include many things dedicated to helping you feel your best. Here are a few ideas that you should be taking a look at:

1. Consider heading out to a restaurant during one of these milestones. You should obviously stick with a Paleo-friendly one. Be sure to do your research.

2. Enjoy an additional Paleo-based dessert.

3. Feel free to skip an exercise period if needed. You should not work out harder than necessary anyway.

4. Enjoy a physical activity with a friend. It can be a nice sports game of any kind. In fact, you should take it easy on yourself for your milestone and stick with a more relaxing kind of sporting activity like bowling or shuffleboard.

These are all very appropriate ways for you to celebrate your milestones while on the diet. They will allow you to not only feel a little more comfortable about your diet but also more likely to go somewhere with it because you will want to reach additional milestones as you go along with it. Your desire to keep on achieving while on the diet should not truly end.

Conclusion

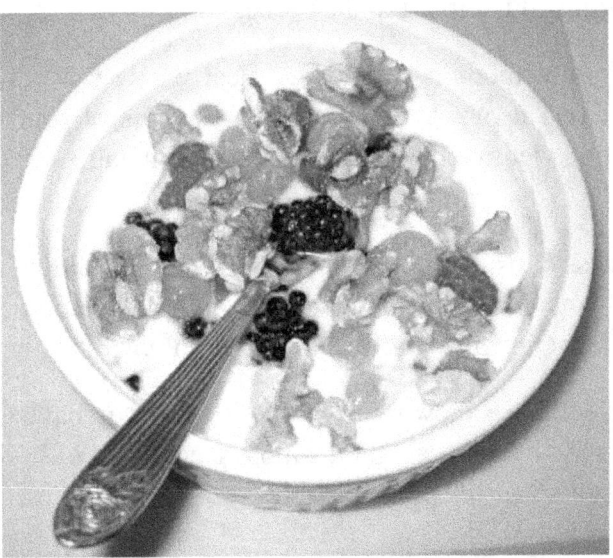

Thanks for reading…how about coconut and berries for a post-guide dessert?

It's completely understandable when a person wonders if the Paleo diet is actually worth it. After all, the unique nature of the diet and the belief behind how it can work are things that some people might question or think differently about. The unique nature of the Paleo diet makes it totally different from other diets.

However, you should have a much easier time with losing weight and getting a healthier body when you do get used to the Paleo diet. You can use the Paleo diet to get your body to be as strong and active as the body of someone who might have been around tens of thousands of years ago.

The brain of the human being has clearly evolved over the years. However, the ways how people are built physically has gone the other way around. People in the Paleolithic Era were able to run well and lift weights and be able to move around the world and survive off of the land. They knew that they had to be healthy and therefore had to focus on the right eating plans to survive.

Meanwhile, today's person has relied on artificial foods and harmful chemicals for far too long. The need to get back in time to focus on a healthier diet and lifestyle has never been more important considering how people are these days.

That's what the concept of the Paleo diet is all about. **It's all to get your body back to nature where it belongs.**

Your diet experience with involve plenty of foods that can work well for weeks or months on end. This can include a good variety of options.

Your experience can also include working with plenty of exercise. This includes not only lifting items but also making sure that your body is controlled with a good level of activity without wearing yourself out in the process.

Naturally, the diet is not without its issues. You clearly have to work hard on the diet in order to stick with it. You also have to be sure that you control yourself as you start out so you can avoid falling victim to the many effects of temptation that the diet can bring about.

Fortunately, the process of using the diet does not have to be all that hard for you to work with. The Paleo diet can be clearly run with the intention of keeping your body active and running well without creating any significant risks with regards to how you might feel.

Hopefully this guide will have shown you everything that you have ever wanted to know about the Paleo diet and how you can get the most success out of it. You can easily use this special diet to get a better lifestyle going.

Remember, eating like a caveman really does have its benefits. It should make you healthier and more likely to lose weight. Just imagine how long one of those cavemen would have lived for had they had access to what we have today while still on the Paleo diet that they had been so used to.